"As a physician who specializes in the treatment of chronic pain syndrome, I can attest to the benefits of engaging in general that ... can ... ease pain. For years I have desired ... clients and patients that was not bulky and complicated. *Essential* ... a practical resource of safe and effective stretches presented in a clear, easy to follow format. Individuals and health care professionals will find this compact guide indispensable in creating and maintaining a general stretching regimen for themselves as well as their clients and patients."

- **Dennis Dobritt, DO, Board Certified - Pain Management & Pain Medicine**

BE SAFE!

The author and publisher of this material are not responsible in any manner whatsoever for any injury that may occur through following the instructions contained in this material. The activities, physical and otherwise, described herein for informational purposes only, may be too strenuous or dangerous for some people and the reader(s) should consult a physician before engaging in them.

motionwise.com

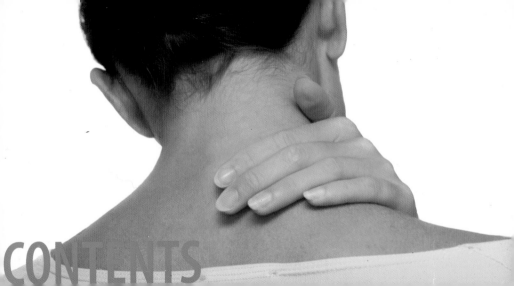

CONTENTS

CONTENTS

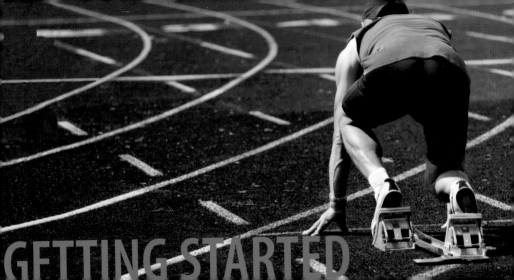

GETTING STARTED

GETTING STARTED

Introduction

If you were married to your muscles, would they stay? One way to take better care of your muscles is to start paying attention to your tension. Muscles that are chronically tight and tense can raise levels of pain and fatigue, and can restrict our ability to move with ease. A general stretching program performed every day is an effective way to exert greater control over your muscular pain, tightness and tension. This book provides support in creating and maintaining a general stretching program. Take a few minutes to stretch every day. Your muscles will thank you.

▶ INSTRUCTIONS

1 Begin by reading the blue pages.

2 Go to your stretch section or the routine section.

3 Learn your stretches and perform your routine on a regular basis.

GETTING STARTED

HEAD NECK

SHOULDER

CHEST

UPPER BACK

ARM, ELBOW HAND

LOWER BACK

HIP

THIGH, KNEE LEG, FOOT

ROUTINES

GETTING STARTED

How can it help to stretch?
Stretching has been reported to increase energy levels, provide greater ease in movement, and increase the efficiency and performance of athletic endeavors.

When should I stretch?
For a general stretching program the best time to stretch is when you will take the time to do it, every day. Although not required, keep in mind that muscles respond most favorably to stretching when they are warm from activities as simple as walking in place or swinging your arms.

How often should I stretch?
We suggest performing a 3 stretch routine 3 times a day, every day. Ask your health care professional for stretch modifications.

Will stretching help my medical condition?
Most doctors and therapists encourage regular stretching. Check with your health care professional to determine if your pain has a muscular component that may be helped by performing selected stretches in this guide.

Should stretching be painful?
To ensure the greatest levels of safety and effectiveness, stretching should not produce pain. You should be able to breathe with comfort, avoid tensing, and remain physically and mentally calm as you stretch. **If pain persists or worsens with stretching, contact your physician.** Some movements may produce non-painful joint noise. Speak to your health care professional before continuing any movement where joint noise is accompanied by pain.

How can I make stretching a habit?

Having a friend or coworker remind you to do your stretches can be very helpful. Also, you can use an activity you do during the day as a reminder to stretch. Every time you make a copy, perform one of your stretches.

How many seconds should I hold a stretch?

This guide advises holding stretches for a number of breaths as opposed to units of time to ensure tension-free stretching.

Won't stress keep tightening my muscles?

Our psychological stresses can increase levels of muscle tightness. Frequent stretching can help reduce levels of muscular tension caused by high levels of stress.

Can stretching enhance my current care?

Stretching can support therapies including physical therapy, chiropractic care and bodywork therapies by helping to keep muscles pliable between sessions. Additionally, engaging in a regular stretching program is an excellent self-care strategy to locate, address and prevent future issues associated with muscular tension.

What are other options for relief?

Talk with your physician or other health care professional about preventative strategies including exercising regularly, using hands-on bodywork, examining areas of psychological stress, and making ergonomic adjustments in your daily activities.

GETTING STARTED

HEAD NECK

SHOULDER

CHEST

UPPER BACK

ARM, ELBOW HAND

LOWER BACK

HIP

THIGH, KNEE LEG, FOOT

ROUTINES

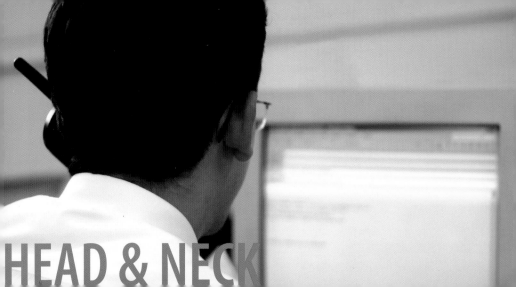

HEAD & NECK

HEAD & NECK

These muscles are tensed by sitting for long periods of time and by extended periods of psychological stress. High risk groups include office and dental professionals, soccer players, cyclists and caregivers.

QUICK START ROUTINES

Zone	Stretch Pages		
Jaw	10	12	16
Head	14	16	38
Neck	14	16	38

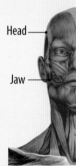
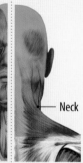

Head

Jaw

Neck

Front View ← → Rear View

GETTING STARTED

HEAD NECK

SHOULDER

CHEST

UPPER BACK

ARM, ELBOW HAND

LOWER BACK

HIP

THIGH, KNEE LEG, FOOT

ROUTINES

FRONTAL NECK STRETCH

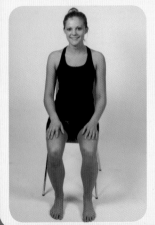
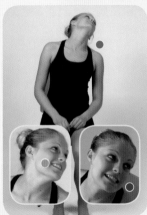

MAY HELP
Headaches
Neck Pain
TMJ (Jaw) Pain

STRETCH TIPS
Keep shoulders relaxed
Teeth together, not clenche
Align front teeth

▶ INSTRUCTIONS

1. Sit comfortably in a stable chair; place front teeth together.
2. Relax head back and rotate to one side.
3. Inhale, exhale and repeat once on the other side.

🔍 This move stretches the platysma muscle which runs from the upper chest to tissue under the chin. This exercise may be performed in a standing or seated position.

GETTING STARTED
HEAD NECK
SHOULDER
CHEST
UPPER BACK
ARM, ELBOW HAND
LOWER BACK
HIP
THIGH, KNEE LEG, FOOT
ROUTINES

JAW STRETCH

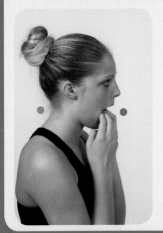
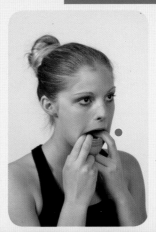

➕ MAY HELP
TMJ (Jaw) Pain
Headaches

✔ STRETCH TIPS
● Let arms hang gently from the jaw
● Head held upright

Essential Stretches - John Gifford

▶ INSTRUCTIONS

1. Relax jaw open and rest the first two fingers of each hand on the lower teeth.
2. Allow the weight of your arms to gently relax the jaw open.
3. Inhale, exhale and repeat once.

This move is most effective in the shower when the muscles are warm. This exercise may be performed in a standing or seated position. Avoid this move if performing it creates discomfort in the jaw.

GETTING STARTED

HEAD NECK

SHOULDER

CHEST

UPPER BACK

ARM, ELBOW HAND

LOWER BACK

HIP

THIGH, KNEE LEG, FOOT

ROUTINES

NECK SERIES

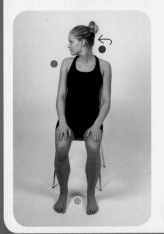

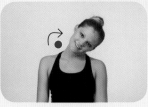

➕ MAY HELP

Headaches

Neck Pain

✔ STRETCH TIPS

- Keep shoulders relaxed
- Feet flat
- Use slow movements

▶ INSTRUCTIONS

1. Sit with feet flat on the floor and hands resting on thighs.
2. Slowly rotate your head from side to side.
3. Return to starting position and slowly tilt head from side to side.
4. Relax head down toward chest and then gently tilt head back. Repeat series three times.

This series of simple movements helps to maintain optimal range of motion in the neck. Speak to your health care professional before continuing any movement where joint noise is accompanied by pain. This exercise may be performed in a standing or seated position.

GETTING STARTED

HEAD NECK

SHOULDER

CHEST

UPPER BACK

ARM, ELBOW HAND

LOWER BACK

HIP

THIGH, KNEE LEG, FOOT

ROUTINES

SEATED NECK STRETCH

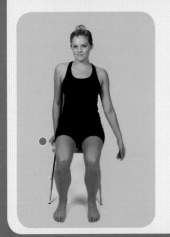 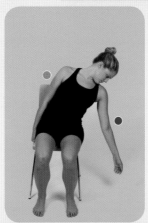

+ MAY HELP
Headaches
Neck Pain
TMJ (Jaw) Pain
Shoulder Pain

✓ STRETCH TIPS
● Firm grasp
● Fully lean to side
● Let arm hang loose

▶ INSTRUCTIONS

1. Sit upright in a chair and grasp the seat with one hand.
2. Slowly lean your body away from grasp, allowing the opposite arm to hang loosely at the side.
3. Relax head down, gazing at your relaxed hand.
4. Inhale, exhale and repeat on the other side.

This move stretches the upper trapezius, a muscle that sits across the top of the shoulder. You may also feel a gentle stretch in the arm grasping the chair.

GETTING STARTED

HEAD NECK

SHOULDER

CHEST

UPPER BACK

ARM, ELBOW HAND

LOWER BACK

HIP

THIGH, KNEE LEG, FOOT

ROUTINES

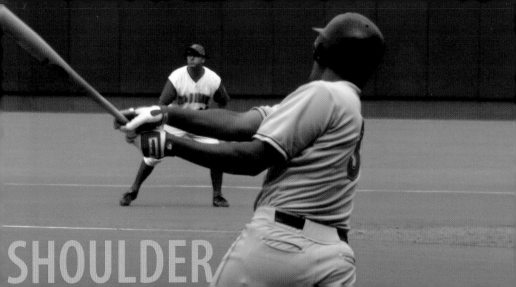

SHOULDER

These muscles are tensed by tasks that require holding arms away from torso, throwing movements, and overhead lifting movements. High risk groups include baseball players, swimmers, painters and dental professionals.

QUICK START ROUTINES

Zone	Stretch Pages		
Front Shoulder	22	30	44
Side Shoulder	22	24	30
Rear Shoulder	20	24	38

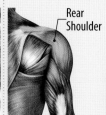

Front Shoulder

Side Shoulder

Rear Shoulder

Front View ⬅➡ Rear View

GETTING STARTED

HEAD NECK

SHOULDER

CHEST

UPPER BACK

ARM, ELBOW HAND

LOWER BACK

HIP

THIGH, KNEE LEG, FOOT

ROUTINES

ARM CROSS STRETCH

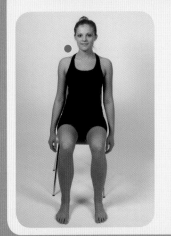
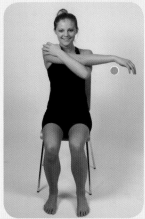

MAY HELP

Shoulder Tension
Upper Back Pain
Rotator Cuff Tension

STRETCH TIPS

Keep shoulders relaxed
Let arm hang loose

▶ INSTRUCTIONS

1. Sit comfortably in a sturdy chair. Reach arm across the body and assist movement by grasping with the opposite arm.
2. Inhale, exhale and repeat twice on each side.

🔍 This move can help relax the rhomboid muscles located between the shoulder blades. This stretch should not produce any discomfort in the front of the shoulder. This exercise may be performed in a standing or seated position.

GETTING STARTED

HEAD NECK

SHOULDER

CHEST

UPPER BACK

ARM, ELBOW HAND

LOWER BACK

HIP

THIGH, KNEE LEG, FOOT

ROUTINES

ARM SWING

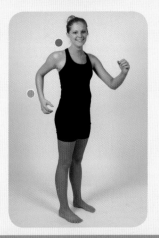

MAY HELP

Shoulder Tension
Upper Back Tension
Neck Pain
Fatigue

✔ **STRETCH TIPS**

● Keep shoulders relaxed
● Let arms hang loose

▶ INSTRUCTIONS

1. Stand with your feet apart, slightly wider than shoulder-width.
2. Freely swing your arms front to back for twelve repetitions.
3. Try to let the arms and hands be free of tension as they swing.

🔍 This is a free-flowing arm swing designed to ease fatigue and tension in the upper back, shoulders and arms. Speak to your health care professional before continuing any movement where joint noise is accompanied by pain.

GETTING STARTED
HEAD NECK
SHOULDER
CHEST
UPPER BACK
ARM, ELBOW HAND
LOWER BACK
HIP
THIGH, KNEE LEG, FOOT
ROUTINES

SHOULDER ROTATION

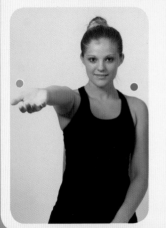
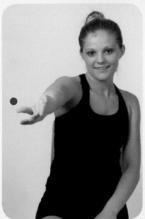

➕ MAY HELP

Shoulder Pain
Arm Pain
Elbow Pain
Rotator Cuff Tension

✓ STRETCH TIPS

● Opposite shoulder relaxed
● Palm facing upwards
● Thumb towards ceiling

▶ INSTRUCTIONS

1. Hold your arm in front of your body with palm facing upwards.
2. Rotate shoulder inward until the thumb is pointing toward the ceiling.
3. Rotate back to starting position.
4. Repeat this cycle four times on each side.

This move can be performed with arm hanging at side to reduce shoulder strain. Speak to your health care professional before continuing any movement where joint noise is accompanied by pain. This exercise may be performed in a standing or seated position.

GETTING STARTED

HEAD NECK

SHOULDER

CHEST

UPPER BACK

ARM, ELBOW HAND

LOWER BACK

HIP

THIGH, KNEE LEG, FOOT

ROUTINES

SHOULDER SHRUG

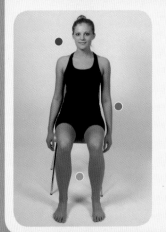
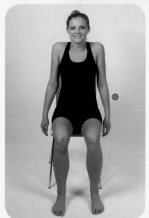

➕ MAY HELP

Shoulder Tension
Upper Back Pain
Headaches

✓ STRETCH TIPS

- Keep arms relaxed
- Legs perpendicular to floor
- Sit tall; don't hunch

▶ INSTRUCTIONS

1. Sit comfortably in a chair with your arms relaxed at your sides.
2. Inhale and raise your shoulders towards your ears.
3. Exhale and let your shoulders return to the starting position.
4. Repeat three times.

🔍 This move can help increase circulation in the trapezius muscle, which can be a source of stiffness when rotating the neck. This exercise may be performed in a standing or seated position.

GETTING STARTED
HEAD NECK
SHOULDER
CHEST
UPPER BACK
ARM, ELBOW HAND
LOWER BACK
HIP
THIGH, KNEE LEG, FOOT
ROUTINES

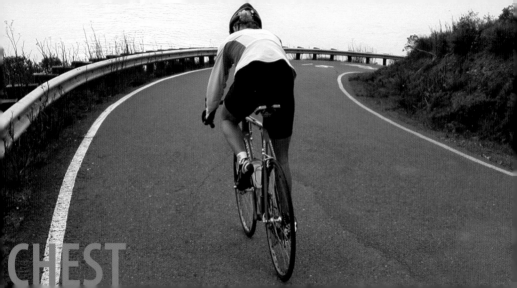

CHEST

CHEST

These muscles are tensed by tasks requiring a hunched forward position, extended periods of carrying, and activities which require moving arms in front of or across body. High risk groups include golf and tennis players, caregivers, runners, office and dental professionals, swimmers, and cyclists.

QUICK START ROUTINE

Zone	Stretch Pages		
Chest	30	32	38

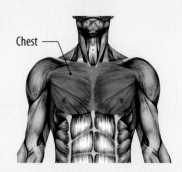

Chest

GETTING STARTED

HEAD NECK

SHOULDER

CHEST

UPPER BACK

ARM, ELBOW HAND

LOWER BACK

HIP

THIGH, KNEE LEG, FOOT

ROUTINES

BACKSTROKE

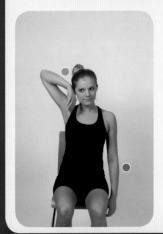 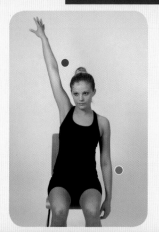

➕ MAY HELP
Rounded Shoulders
Neck Pain
Shoulder Pain
Upper Back Pain

✔ STRETCH TIPS
● Keep arm relaxed at side
● Wrist to ear
● Elbow extended

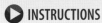

▶ INSTRUCTIONS

1. Sit with feet shoulder-width apart.
2. Place wrist to ear, then reach up and back in a circle as if doing the backstroke in water.
3. Repeat four to eight times on each side, switching sides between repetitions.

This move can relax the chest muscles, allowing better posture and reduced tension in the shoulders and upper back. Speak to your health care professional before continuing any movement where joint noise is accompanied by pain. This exercise may be performed in a standing or seated position.

GETTING STARTED

HEAD NECK

SHOULDER

CHEST

UPPER BACK

ARM, ELBOW HAND

LOWER BACK

HIP

THIGH, KNEE LEG, FOOT

ROUTINES

DOORWAY CHEST STRETCH

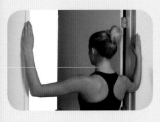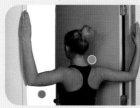

+ MAY HELP
Rounded Shoulders
Shoulder Pain
Upper Back Pain
Arm Pain

✓ STRETCH TIPS
- Keep upper arms parallel to floor
- Keep neck relaxed

▶ INSTRUCTIONS

1. Stand in doorway with feet shoulder-width apart.
2. Place your hands on either side of the door opening.
   You can position elbows slightly higher than shoulders to reduce shoulder strain.
3. Slowly relax your body forward.
4. Inhale, exhale and repeat once.

🔍 Keeping the chest relaxed can actually help improve posture and relieve upper back tension. Avoid this stretch if you feel any level of discomfort in the shoulders or the lower back.

GETTING STARTED
HEAD NECK
SHOULDER
CHEST
UPPER BACK
ARM, ELBOW HAND
LOWER BACK
HIP
THIGH, KNEE LEG, FOOT
ROUTINES

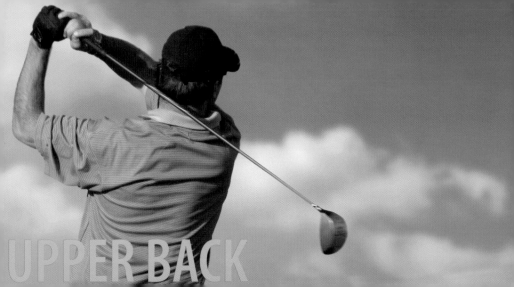

UPPER BACK

UPPER BACK

These muscles are tensed by carrying heavy items and by extended periods of sitting. High risk groups include swimmers, gardeners, golf players, and office professionals.

QUICK START ROUTINES

Zone	Stretch Pages		
Between Shoulder Blades	20	30	38
On Shoulder Blade	20	22	24

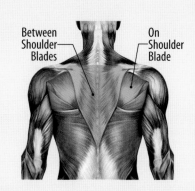

Between Shoulder Blades

On Shoulder Blade

GETTING STARTED

HEAD NECK

SHOULDER

CHEST

UPPER BACK

ARM, ELBOW HAND

LOWER BACK

HIP

THIGH, KNEE LEG, FOOT

ROUTINES

CAT BACK

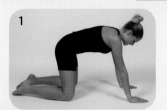

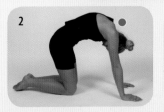

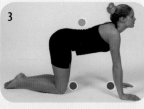

➕ MAY HELP

Upper Back Pain
Neck Tightness
Shoulder Tightness
Lower Back Tension

✔ STRETCH TIPS

● Neck & shoulders relaxed
● Let back relax
● Thighs & forearms perpendicular to floor

▶ INSTRUCTIONS

1. Position your body on hands and knees, with knees slightly wider than hip-width apart.
2. Slowly inhale as you raise your upper back and relax head down.
3. Exhale and let your lower back relax down as you raise your head.
4. Perform four repetitions.

🔍 This move helps reduce tension in the group of spinal muscles which span from the lower back up to the base of the skull.

GETTING STARTED

HEAD NECK

SHOULDER

CHEST

UPPER BACK

ARM, ELBOW HAND

LOWER BACK

HIP

THIGH, KNEE LEG, FOOT

ROUTINES

ROUNDED SHOULDER STRETCH

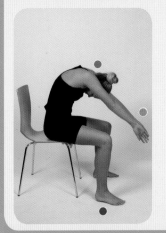
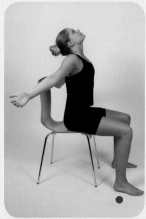

MAY HELP

Upper Back Pain
Shoulder Pain
Improve Posture

STRETCH TIPS

Keep head relaxed
Backs of hands touch
Feet flat on floor

Essential Stretches - John Gifford

▶ INSTRUCTIONS

1. Sit on the edge of your chair with your knees apart.
2. Relax your head down, round the upper back, rotate your shoulders and arms so that the backs of your hands touch.
3. Open your arms back, let your head move up and back as you rotate your shoulders open with your palms facing upward.
4. Relax arms at side and repeat sequence four times.

🔍 This move engages the muscles of the chest and upper back. Speak to your health care professional before continuing any movement where joint noise is accompanied by pain. This exercise may be performed in a standing or seated position.

GETTING STARTED

HEAD NECK

SHOULDER

CHEST

UPPER BACK

ARM, ELBOW HAND

LOWER BACK

HIP

THIGH, KNEE LEG, FOOT

ROUTINES

THREAD THE NEEDLE

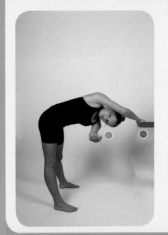

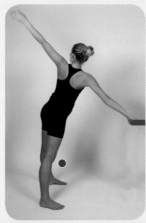

⊕ MAY HELP

Upper Back Pain
Lower Back Pain
Shoulder Tension

✓ STRETCH TIPS

● Stationary support
● Eyes follow hand
● Keep knees straight

GETTING STARTED

HEAD NECK

SHOULDER

CHEST

UPPER BACK

ARM, ELBOW HAND

LOWER BACK

HIP

THIGH, KNEE LEG, FOOT

ROUTINES

▶ INSTRUCTIONS

1. Stand with feet shoulder-width apart, one hand grasping a stationary support.
2. Reach one hand under your body, allowing your head to rotate.
3. Reach your arm as far as comfortable in the opposite direction.
4. Repeat three times using continuous motion and switch to other side.

🔍 This move can help relieve tension in the muscles responsible for the rotation of the lumbar spine. Speak to your health care professional before continuing any movement where joint noise is accompanied by pain.

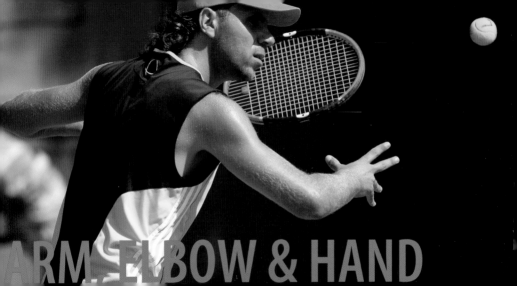

ARM, ELBOW & HAND

ARM, ELBOW & HAND

These muscles are tensed by activities that require gripping, wrist rotation, and repetitive finger movement. High risk groups include tennis, golf, piano and guitar players, dental and computer professionals.

QUICK START ROUTINES

Zone	Stretch Pages		
Bicep Region	30	38	44
Elbow Area	24	30	46
Wrist & Hand	24	30	48
Tricep Area	24	30	46

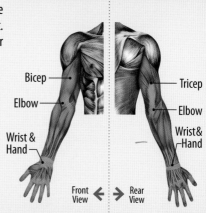

Bicep

Elbow

Wrist & Hand

Tricep

Elbow

Wrist & Hand

Front View ← → Rear View

GETTING STARTED

HEAD NECK

SHOULDER

CHEST

UPPER BACK

ARM, ELBOW HAND

LOWER BACK

HIP

THIGH, KNEE LEG, FOOT

ROUTINES

BICEP STRETCH

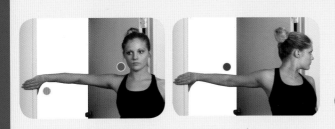

+ MAY HELP
Arm Pain
Tennis Elbow
Shoulder Pain

✓ STRETCH TIPS
● Shoulder relaxed down
● Thumb pointing down
● Elbow straight

Essential Stretches - John Gifford

▶ INSTRUCTIONS

1. Stand next to a door jamb, grasping door frame with your thumb pointing down.
2. Slowly turn your upper body away from the door frame until you feel a gentle stretch in the upper arm.
3. Inhale, exhale and repeat on other arm.

🔍 This move stretches the bicep muscle which lies on the front of the upper arm and may help relieve shoulder pain and tennis elbow.

GETTING STARTED

HEAD NECK

SHOULDER

CHEST

UPPER BACK

ARM, ELBOW HAND

LOWER BACK

HIP

THIGH, KNEE LEG, FOOT

ROUTINES

TRICEP STRETCH

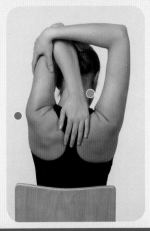

➕ MAY HELP

Elbow Pain

Arm Pain

Shoulder Pain

✔ STRETCH TIPS

● Keep shoulders relaxed

● Let neck relax forward

▶ INSTRUCTIONS

1. Sit comfortably in a chair.
2. Reach one hand behind your head to the upper back.
3. Place other hand on top of the elbow and pull as far as comfortable.
4. Inhale, exhale and repeat on the other side.

🔍 This move stretches the largest muscle in the back of the upper arm, the tricep, and can help relax the shoulders. This exercise may be performed in a standing or seated position.

GETTING STARTED

HEAD NECK

SHOULDER

CHEST

UPPER BACK

ARM, ELBOW HAND

LOWER BACK

HIP

THIGH, KNEE LEG, FOOT

ROUTINES

WRIST RELIEVER

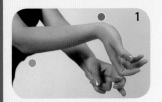
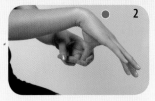
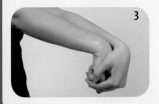
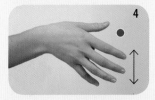

➕ MAY HELP
Hand Pain
Tennis Elbow
Wrist Pain

✔ STRETCH TIPS
● Let wrist relax down
● Keep elbow bent
● Shake hand

Essential Stretches - John Gifford

▶ INSTRUCTIONS

1. Stretch each finger back towards your elbow.
2. Turn hand over and stretch thumb back.
3. Place one hand on top of the other and curl fingers under.
4. Shake hand briefly and repeat on other hand.

🔍 Perform all portions of this series slowly and gently to avoid creating any discomfort in the wrist, fingers or thumb. This exercise may be performed in a standing or seated position.

GETTING STARTED
HEAD NECK
SHOULDER
CHEST
UPPER BACK
ARM, ELBOW HAND
LOWER BACK
HIP
THIGH, KNEE LEG, FOOT
ROUTINES

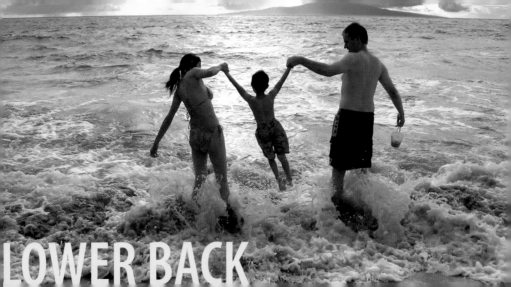

LOWER BACK

LOWER BACK

These muscles are tensed by extended periods of sitting or bent-over postures, tasks that require lifting, activities requiring lateral movements, and extended periods of psychological stress. High risk groups include golf, tennis, hockey, and racquetball players, office professionals, and caregivers.

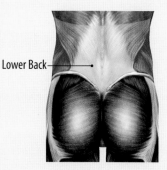

Lower Back

QUICK START ROUTINES

Series	Stretch Pages		
Standing Series	60	74	84
Seated Series	56	68	82
Floor Series	52	54	58

GETTING STARTED

HEAD NECK

SHOULDER

CHEST

UPPER BACK

ARM, ELBOW HAND

LOWER BACK

HIP

THIGH, KNEE LEG, FOOT

ROUTINES

LOWER BACK STRETCH

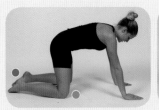 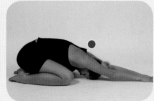

+ MAY HELP
Lower Back Pain
Shoulder Tightness
Hip Tension
Upper Back Tension

✔ STRETCH TIPS
● Ankles close together
● Knees hip width apart
● Keep neck, shoulders
& chest relaxed

Essential Stretches - John Gifford

▶ INSTRUCTIONS

1. Position your body on hands and knees, with knees slightly wider than hip width apart. Move feet in slightly allowing lower legs to angle inward.
2. Lower hips back towards ankles as you slowly walk hands forward as far as comfortable, letting head relax down.
3. Inhale, exhale five times and walk hands back to starting position.

This move gently stretches the lower back muscles which can also help relieve tension in the upper back and shoulders. Avoid this move if it causes discomfort in the groin, knees or ankles.

GETTING STARTED

HEAD NECK

SHOULDER

CHEST

UPPER BACK

ARM, ELBOW HAND

LOWER BACK

HIP

THIGH, KNEE LEG, FOOT

ROUTINES

LYING SPINAL ROTATION

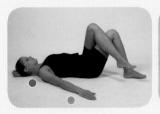 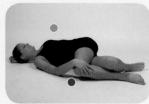

+ MAY HELP

Lower Back Pain
Upper Back Pain
Hip Pain
Sciatica

✔ STRETCH TIPS

● Keep neck, shoulders
& chest relaxed

● Arms away from body

● Let gravity guide the
movement, not force

Essential Stretches - John Gifford

▶ INSTRUCTIONS

1. Lie on your back with your left knee crossed over your right knee.
2. Place your right hand on the left knee and let gravity guide your knees down towards the floor.
3. Inhale, exhale four times and return to the starting position.
4. Cross the right knee over the left knee; repeat on the opposite side.

This move gently rotates the lower spine, stretching the deep muscles of the lower back and the hips. Speak to your health care professional before continuing any movement where joint noise is accompanied by pain.

GETTING STARTED

HEAD NECK

SHOULDER

CHEST

UPPER BACK

ARM, ELBOW HAND

LOWER BACK

HIP

THIGH, KNEE LEG, FOOT

ROUTINES

LYING SPINAL ROTATION

SIDE-BENDING STRETCH

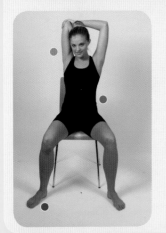
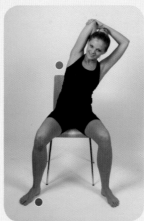

➕ MAY HELP
Lower Back Pain
Shoulder Pain
Hip Pain

✔ STRETCH TIPS
● Sit tall; don't hunch
● Keep neck relaxed
● Feet flat on the floor

▶ INSTRUCTIONS

1. Place one hand on the upper back and the other hand on the elbow.
2. Bend to the side of the hand on the elbow until you feel a stretch.
3. Inhale and exhale, trying to relax further into the stretch.
4. Return to starting position and repeat sequence on the other side.

This move can help release tension in the muscles located on the side of the torso from the top of the hip up to the shoulder blade.

GETTING STARTED

HEAD NECK

SHOULDER

CHEST

UPPER BACK

ARM, ELBOW HAND

LOWER BACK

HIP

THIGH, KNEE LEG, FOOT

ROUTINES

SIDE-LYING STRETCH

+ MAY HELP
Lower Back Pain
Hip Pain
Sciatica

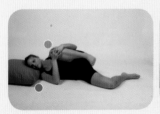
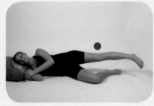

✔ STRETCH TIPS
● Support head
● Knee towards shoulder
● Extend knee

Essential Stretches - John Gifford

▶ INSTRUCTIONS

1. Lie on your side with your head supported and knees flexed.
2. Using both arms, gently bring the top knee towards your shoulder.
3. Slowly extend the knee and return to starting position.
4. Repeat four times on each side.

This move can help relax the hip and lower back muscles, releasing tension in the lower back. The side-lying position adds to the safety of this stretch. Discontinue this move if performing it generates any discomfort in the groin.

GETTING STARTED

HEAD NECK

SHOULDER

CHEST

UPPER BACK

ARM, ELBOW HAND

LOWER BACK

HIP

THIGH, KNEE LEG, FOOT

ROUTINES

STANDING BACK STRETCH

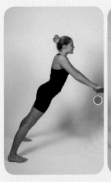 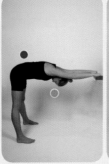 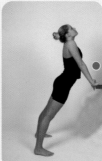

+ MAY HELP
Back & Hip Pain
Shoulder Tension
Tight Hamstrings

✔ STRETCH TIPS

● Stationary support & elbows straight

● Let head hang freely

● Flatten lower back

▶ INSTRUCTIONS

1. Stand arms length away from a stationary support.
2. Grasp support and move feet apart, slightly wider than shoulder-width.
3. Flatten lower back. Slowly move hips away from support, letting your head hang down. Inhale, exhale.
4. Move hips towards support. As your back straightens let head relax back.
5. Inhale, exhale and step towards support before releasing grasp.

🔍 You may feel stretching in the hamstring and calf muscles located on the back of the thigh and leg, as well as hip flexors located in the front of the pelvis and upper thigh. Discontinue this move if performing it generates any discomfort in the lower back.

GETTING STARTED

HEAD NECK

SHOULDER

CHEST

UPPER BACK

ARM, ELBOW HAND

LOWER BACK

HIP

THIGH, KNEE LEG, FOOT

ROUTINES

STANDING BACK STRETCH

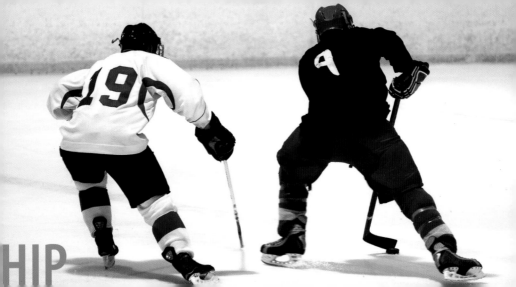

HIP

These muscles are tensed by side-to-side or repetitive hip movements, lifting items from ground level, extended periods of sitting, or psychological stress. High risk groups include hockey and tennis players, cyclists, dancers, and office professionals.

QUICK START ROUTINES

Zone	Stretch Pages		
Side Of Hip	54	58	64
Hip Flexors/Groin	66	74	84
Gluteal	58	64	68

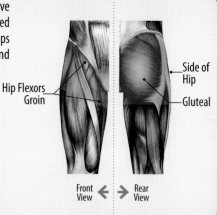

Hip Flexors
Groin

Side of Hip

Gluteal

Front View ← → Rear View

GETTING STARTED
HEAD NECK
SHOULDER
CHEST
UPPER BACK
ARM, ELBOW HAND
LOWER BACK
HIP
THIGH, KNEE LEG, FOOT
ROUTINES

CROSS HIP STRETCH

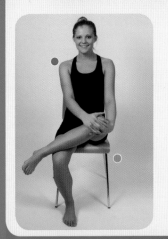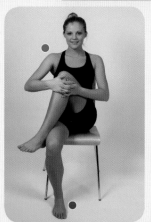

➕ MAY HELP
Hip Pain
Sciatica
Lower Back Pain

✔ STRETCH TIPS
● Keep shoulders relaxed
● Stable chair - no wheels!
● Foot flat on floor

▶ INSTRUCTIONS

1. Place one leg on top of the opposite thigh.
2. Interlock fingers over the knee as shown.
3. Guide knee in the direction of the opposite shoulder.
4. Inhale, exhale and repeat on the other side.

This move can help relax the gluteal muscles on the side of the hip, which can in turn release tension in the lower back. Discontinue this move if performing it generates any discomfort in the groin.

GETTING STARTED

HEAD NECK

SHOULDER

CHEST

UPPER BACK

ARM, ELBOW HAND

LOWER BACK

HIP

THIGH, KNEE LEG, FOOT

ROUTINES

KNEELING HIP FLEXOR

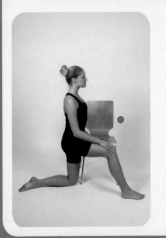
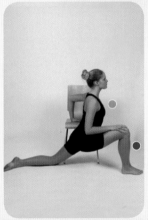

+ MAY HELP

Hip Pain
Sciatica
Lower Back Pain

✓ STRETCH TIPS

● Stable chair - no wheels!
● Maintain upright posture
● Leg perpendicular to floor

▶ INSTRUCTIONS

1. Kneel beside a chair, placing one hand on the seat of the chair and the other on top of the thigh.
2. Slowly move your body forward until you feel a stretch in the front of the hip closest to the chair. Inhale, exhale three times.
3. Turn to face the opposite direction and repeat on the other side.

🔍 This move can help relax the hip flexor muscles which are located in the front of the pelvis and upper thigh, releasing tension in the lower back.

GETTING STARTED

HEAD NECK

SHOULDER

CHEST

UPPER BACK

ARM, ELBOW HAND

LOWER BACK

HIP

THIGH, KNEE LEG, FOOT

ROUTINES

SEATED HIP STRETCH

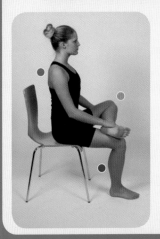
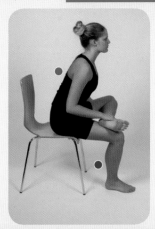

➕ **MAY HELP**
- Hip Pain
- Sciatica
- Lower Back Pain
- Leg Pain

✔️ **STRETCH TIPS**
- 🔴 Sit tall & relaxed
- 🟢 Hand under knee
- ⚫ Leg perpendicular to floor

▶ INSTRUCTIONS

1. Place one ankle on top of the opposite knee.
2. Place one hand on the ankle and cradle knee with other hand.
3. Slowly lean your body forward while keeping your back straight and lifting your knee slightly towards your chest.
4. Inhale, exhale and repeat on the other side.

This move can help relax the piriformis, a deep hip muscle, which can be a critical muscle for sciatica sufferers. Remember to place hand under, not on, top of the knee.

GETTING STARTED

HEAD NECK

SHOULDER

CHEST

UPPER BACK

ARM, ELBOW HAND

LOWER BACK

HIP

THIGH, KNEE LEG, FOOT

ROUTINES

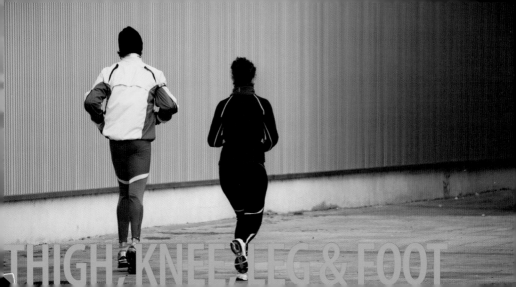

THIGH, KNEE, LEG & FOOT

THIGH, KNEE, LEG & FOOT

These muscles are tensed by extended periods of sitting and standing, activities with high levels of start and stop movements, and tasks requiring hunched-over posture while standing. High risk groups include golf, hockey and tennis players, cyclists, runners, and office professionals.

QUICK START ROUTINES

Zone		Stretch Pages		
Thigh & Knee	Front	66	68	84
	Back	60	80	82
	Inside	58	66	74
	Outside	54	64	74

Zone		Stretch Pages		
Lower Leg	Calf	76	80	82
	Shin	72	76	80
	Foot	72	76	80

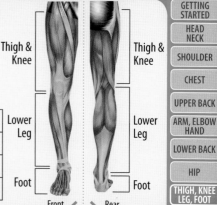

Thigh & Knee

Thigh & Knee

Lower Leg

Lower Leg

Foot

Foot

Front View

Rear View

GETTING STARTED

HEAD NECK

SHOULDER

CHEST

UPPER BACK

ARM, ELBOW HAND

LOWER BACK

HIP

THIGH, KNEE LEG, FOOT

ROUTINES

FOOT STRETCH

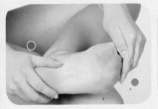 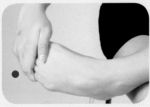

➕ MAY HELP
Foot Pain
Ankle Pain
Plantar Fasciitis
Foot Cramps

✔ STRETCH TIPS
- Support Heel
- Grasp bottom of toes
- Place hand on top of toes

Essential Stretches - John Gifford

▷ **INSTRUCTIONS**

1. Sitting in a chair, place ankle on thigh. Support heel and stretch toes back towards the knee. Inhale, exhale.
2. Move hand from heel to the top of the toes.
3. Extend ankle and stretch the top of the toes away from the knee.
4. Inhale, exhale and repeat sequence on the other side.

🔍 This move targets the often neglected muscles of the feet. It can be particularly helpful in reducing nighttime cramping of the foot and toes.

GETTING STARTED

HEAD NECK

SHOULDER

CHEST

UPPER BACK

ARM, ELBOW HAND

LOWER BACK

HIP

THIGH, KNEE LEG, FOOT

ROUTINES

HIP WAGS

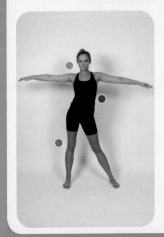
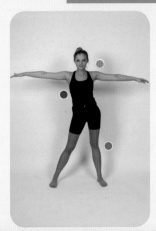

➕ MAY HELP

Inner Thigh Tightness
Knee Pain
Lower Back Pain
Hip Tightness

✔ STRETCH TIPS

- Keep knees straight
- Keep shoulders level
- Maintain upright posture

Essential Stretches - John Gifford

▶ INSTRUCTIONS

1. Begin with feet placed slightly wider than shoulder-width.
   You may grasp a stable, non-wheeled chair for support.
2. Keeping the knees straight, gently shift your hips from side to side.
3. For a greater stretch, move feet as far apart as comfortable.
4. Repeat four times.

This movement is designed to gently stretch the adductors, the muscles of the inner thigh. Tight inner thigh muscles can contribute to knee and lower back pain.

GETTING STARTED
HEAD NECK
SHOULDER
CHEST
UPPER BACK
ARM, ELBOW HAND
LOWER BACK
HIP
THIGH, KNEE LEG, FOOT
ROUTINES

KNEE BENDS

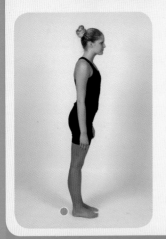
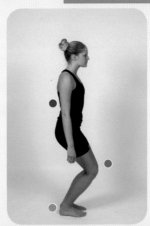

➕ MAY HELP

Calf Cramps
Knee Pain
Lower Back Pain
Hip Pain

✅ STRETCH TIPS

- Keep knees together
- Keep heels flat
- Maintain upright posture

Essential Stretches - John Gifford

▶ INSTRUCTIONS

1. **Stand tall with your feet and knees together.**
   You may grasp a stable, non-wheeled chair for support.

2. **Bend knees slightly, keeping feet flat on the floor.**

3. **Return to standing position.**

4. **Perform four to eight times.**

Perform this simple movement to help ease tension in the lower body, especially when standing for long periods of time. Speak to your health care professional before continuing any movement where joint noise is accompanied by pain.

GETTING STARTED

HEAD NECK

SHOULDER

CHEST

UPPER BACK

ARM, ELBOW HAND

LOWER BACK

HIP

THIGH, KNEE LEG, FOOT

ROUTINES

LYING HAMSTRING & CALF STRETCH

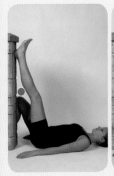 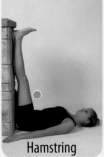 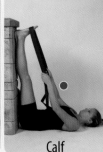

Hamstring

Calf

➕ MAY HELP

Tight Hamstrings
Calf Tightness & Cramps
Knee Pain
Lower Back Pain

✔ STRETCH TIPS

● Opposite knee bent
● Keep thigh relaxed
● Let arms hang gently

Essential Stretches - John Gifford

▶ INSTRUCTIONS

1. Lie on the floor and place one foot on an upright support, such as a door frame, while keeping the other knee bent.

2. Move hips towards the support until you feel a gentle stretch in your hamstrings (back of thigh). Inhale, exhale five times and repeat on other side.

3. To target your calf muscles place a strap, towel or sheet over the ball of your foot, and let your arms hang gently as they grasp the strap. Inhale, exhale five times and repeat on the other side.

This approach targets the hamstring and calf muscles, located on the back of the leg and thigh, while keeping the lower back supported and safe.

GETTING STARTED

HEAD NECK

SHOULDER

CHEST

UPPER BACK

ARM, ELBOW HAND

LOWER BACK

HIP

THIGH, KNEE LEG, FOOT

ROUTINES

SEATED CALF STRETCH

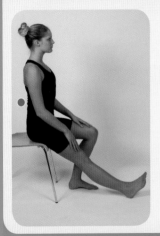 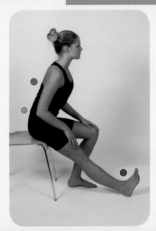

➕ MAY HELP

Calf Tightness
Plantar Fasciitis
Lower Back Pain
Knee Pain
Ankle Tightness

✔ STRETCH TIPS

● Sit tall; don't hunch
● Bend from the waist
● Flex ankle & toes back

▶ INSTRUCTIONS

1. Sit tall in a chair with one leg extended and a hand on each thigh.
2. Flex the ankle of the extended leg back toward your torso.
3. Bending at the waist, move forward until you feel a mild stretch in the calf muscle located behind the knee.
4. Inhale, exhale and repeat on the other side.

🔍 Tightness in the gastrocnemius, a calf muscle located behind the knee, can be a hidden contributor to foot cramps, as well as tension in the knee, ankle, and even the lower back.

GETTING STARTED

HEAD NECK

SHOULDER

CHEST

UPPER BACK

ARM, ELBOW HAND

LOWER BACK

HIP

THIGH, KNEE LEG, FOOT

ROUTINES

SEATED CALF STRETCH

SEATED HAMSTRING STRETCH

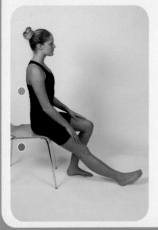 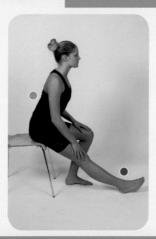

➕ MAY HELP

Tight Hamstrings
Knee Pain
Lower Back Pain
Sciatica

✔ STRETCH TIPS

● Stable chair - no wheels!
● Sit tall; don't hunch
● Keep ankle relaxed

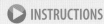 **INSTRUCTIONS**

1. Sit tall in a stable, non-wheeled chair with one leg extended.
2. Place one hand on each thigh.
3. Slowly bend at the waist until you feel a gentle stretch in the hamstring muscles located on the back of the thigh.
4. Inhale, exhale and repeat on the other side.

This move lengthens the hamstrings, a muscle group located on the back of the thigh, which can contribute to lower back pain.

GETTING STARTED

HEAD NECK

SHOULDER

CHEST

UPPER BACK

ARM, ELBOW HAND

LOWER BACK

HIP

THIGH, KNEE LEG, FOOT

ROUTINES

STANDING THIGH STRETCH

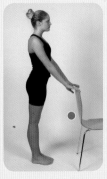
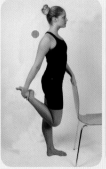
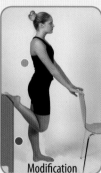

Modification

➕ MAY HELP

Knee Pain
Lower Back Pain
Hip Pain
Tight Hip Flexors

✅ STRETCH TIPS

- Stable chair - no wheels!
- Maintain upright posture
- Stationary foot support

▶ INSTRUCTIONS

1. Stand with feet hip-width apart, holding a stable support.
2. Hold on to the back of the chair with your left hand and bring your right foot to your right hand to create a mild stretch.
   Support your foot on a bed or couch for greater ease and added stability.
3. Inhale, exhale and repeat on the other side.

🔍 This move can help relax the quadricep and hip flexor muscles located in the front of the pelvis and upper thigh, releasing tension in the lower back. Avoid this move if it generates discomfort in the knee or cramping in the back of thigh.

GETTING STARTED

HEAD NECK

SHOULDER

CHEST

UPPER BACK

ARM, ELBOW HAND

LOWER BACK

HIP

THIGH, KNEE LEG, FOOT

ROUTINES

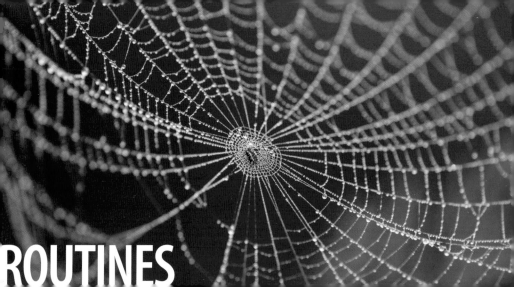

ROUTINES

ROUTINES

Choose from these standard stretching routines or turn the page to create your own.

General Wellness	Stretch Pages			Your Activity	Stretch Pages		
Monday	22	24	30	Sitting	16	68	84
Tuesday	68	80	82	Standing	74	80	82
Wednesday	26	38	56	Kneeling & Bending	32	44	60
Thursday	14	16	20	Walking	60	74	84
Friday	40	60	74	Fine Motor (Hands)	38	44	48
Saturday	52	54	58	Upper Body Sport	16	30	38
Sunday	54	66	78	Lower Body Sport	66	68	78

GETTING STARTED

HEAD NECK

SHOULDER

CHEST

UPPER BACK

ARM, ELBOW HAND

LOWER BACK

HIP

THIGH, KNEE LEG, FOOT

ROUTINES

CREATE YOUR OWN ROUTINE

Before You Begin

When creating your routine, keep in mind that different muscles can affect one another like the strands of a spider web. Muscular pain can be impacted by the muscles directly located around a pain area or by related muscles pulling from a distance. ●**DIRECT STRETCHES** are those stretches that directly target your specific area of need. ○**RELATED STRETCHES** can indirectly help with pain and tension in your specific area by relaxing remote areas of tightness. For example, performing stretches in the HIP section may aid in relaxing the LOWER BACK.

▶ INSTRUCTIONS

1 Choose your section in the stretch index.

2 Choose 3 stretches from your section row.

3 Perform your routine 3 times a day.